Untold Secret of Overcoming

EBOLA

The Ultimate Guide to Living a Healthy Free-Ebola Lifestyle

By Mike Okonkwo

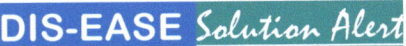

DIS-EASE *Solution Alert*

...bringing people back to peaceful and happy life; free from Fear & Stress of Ebola Sickness

Untold Secret of Overcoming
EBOLA

The Ultimate Guide to Living a Healthy Free-Ebola Lifestyle

ISBN -13: 978-1502330406

Untold Secret of Overcoming EBOLA -

(The Ultimate Guide to Living a Healthy Free-Ebola Lifestyle)

By
GYCD Initiative/GOOD HEALTH CENTER
www.gycdi.com

Book Concept + Production
CCN Concepts
+234 (0) 805 9813 579
Email: ccnconsultants@yahoo.com

Acknowledgements

I0435242

Every form of accomplishment in life is as result of contribution and corporate support of many people in our lives. This work is no different. I want to thank my close friend and IT Consultant Mr. Kola Abdulsalam who continues to encourage me to put my thoughts in print believing it will benefit the global community. Consultant Kola, your motivation, contribution and follow-up made this project possible for me to deliver this manuscript to the world.

Many thanks to my wife, Sharon Okonkwo, my son and friend Bobby Michael Greenfields and Somto Great who allowed and supported me to spend nights and days researching and staring at my laptop screen to produce this book

To my father in faith and mentor Apostle H.I. Alile OFR; Senior colleague, Rev Moses Olowoporoku and associates, Pastor Uche Chris, Pastor Ugo Adimibe, Elder Andi Iwuanynwu, Dcn. Okey Odunze, Dcn. Gbenga Olugbenle, Dcn Onuoha Kachi, Pastor Victor Mukwuzi, Sunny Omole, Kingsley Odili and Samuel Francis who believe so much in me that I can deliver and motivated me. My appreciation to you all is beyond words.

To all the staff, members and visitors of Good Health Center, this book is as result of your faith in me as your Executive Director and your questions that forced me to seek answers to Ebola issues that needed addressing. Thank you all.

The most important thanks go to God for inspiration and capability to write this book.

About GOOD HEALTH CENTER

The GOOD HEALTH CENTER was established by **Grassroots Youth Capacity Development Initiative**, as a nonprofit, charitable, Non-Governmental Organization; passionately devoted to serving the African people through the facilitation of personal discovery and motivational development of Biblical pathways leading to building health and fighting degenerative diseases.

Mission
- To help African community acquire optimal health and wellness through education, instructional programs, and trainings.
- To provide supports that lead to disease prevention and reversal strategies.
- To produce or support production of affordable healthy foods and health & lifestyle services.

Core Values
- We believe that God created human beings as Spirit, Soul and Body, each part integrally related, identifiably separate but in communication with each other; and combining to facilitate the potential achievement of optimal health and wellness.
- We believe to achieve optimal health and wellness every aspect of all the other segments of life will be touched.
- We believe God divinely created every individual with the God given birthright and entitled to prerogative right of optimal health and wellness.

Operational Structure
- We conduct weekly free health building and disease fighting Seminars at various locations in Nigeria.

- We hold seminars and workshops for groups and individuals in collaboration with churches, Ministries, Agencies, Institutions, Corporate bodies and Governments.
- We publish nutritionally based health building and disease fighting books and journals,
- We distribute and sometimes produce healthy foods to those with health challenge.
- We are willing to collaborate with international and local donors agencies.

Disclaimer

All content and information in this Book, our manuals and Seminars are for general informational purposes only. They are not intended to be a substitute for the advice, diagnosis, or treatment of a qualified Medical doctor or practitioner. All matters regarding your health require medical supervision. Neither the publisher nor the authors shall be liable or responsible for any loss or damage allegedly arising from any information or suggestion in this Manual.

However, the Publisher does encourage the sharing and careful review of the information contained in this Manual with one's professional health care provider.

Introduction

Ebola dis-ease of pandemic in Africa is now a World Health issue because of the high contagious nature of the disease and increasing death rate. An infected person can easily transfer Ebola to a whole nation just by mere visit to that nation. For instance only one man from Liberia visited Nigeria. In a space of one month Ebola became a national problem in Nigeria.

Because of the devastating effect of Ebola, a public affairs analyst said, at the rate Ebola is spreading in West Africa, if no constructive and serious measure is taken to curb it now, Africa may be losing more lives than Nigeria is losing from Boko Haram attacks. *(Boko haram is a terrorist group operating in Nigeria)* This translates to mean that Ebola is adjudged more deadly than terrorists, ethnic and religious wars in Africa.

Another challenge is that the Governments of the affected nations in Africa and their professional groups responsible for scientific medicine and administration seem to be powerless as they have told us that Ebola has no known cure for now. What can we say is happening to our health care system? Is the law of diminishing returns setting in that the more they put into it the less it becomes effective?

The media hype on Ebola to inform citizens the dangers of Ebola seem to been causing more deaths by injecting fear in the people. Through same media we learned that as the medical industry claimed no solution some people offered unsolicited and unapproved salt therapy. Some tried it as preventive measure and died. A radio commentator said "the fear of Ebola can kill faster than the Ebola disease itself".

In times like this where is God? I am confident that in times like this God the creator of man will not leave the people comfortless. He has promised to restore our health and heal our wounds and that His recommended foods for man will become our medicine for the healing of the nations. (Jer. 30:17; Gen. 1:29; Rev.12:2).

Based on the words of the Manufacturer (God), I totally disagree that Ebola has no cure hence I agree with Dr. Alexis Carrel's 1936 prediction - *"unless the doctors of today become the dieticians of tomorrow, the dieticians of today will become the doctors of tomorrow"*

THE EBOLA DISEASE

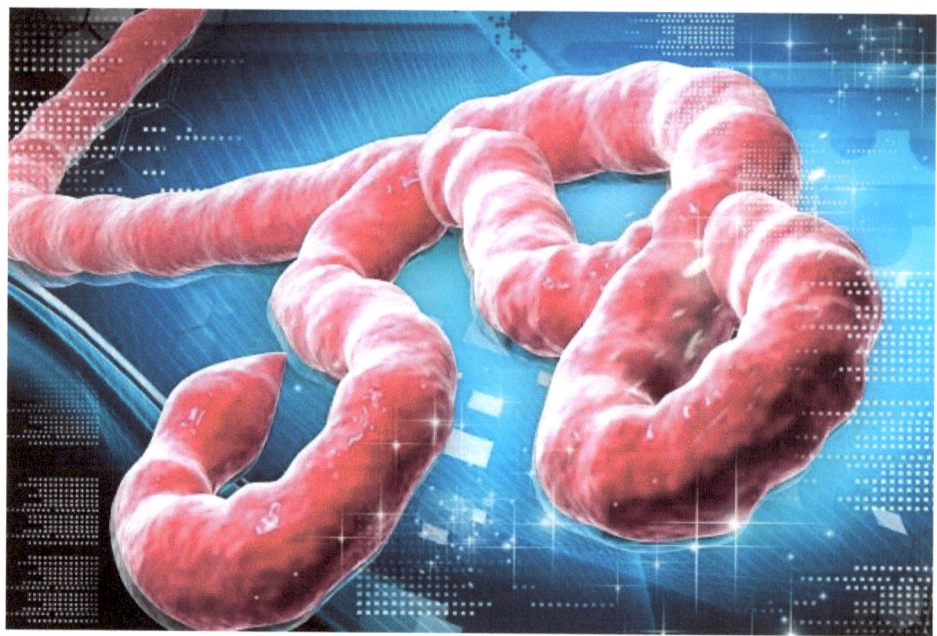

There have been different views and write-ups on Ebola disease, which is now ravaging some parts of Africa and gradually creeping into Europe and America. Strange Acts Today, Vol.1 No 32 writes "Ebola Virus disease (EVD) or Ebola Hemorrhagic Fever (EHF) is the human disease caused by the Ebola virus. Symptoms typically start two days to three weeks after contracting the virus..."

"This emerging health threat is the result of a RNA (ribonucleic acid) virus that infects wild animals — like fruit bats, monkeys, gorillas, and chimpanzees — as well as people. Contact with an infected animal's blood or body fluids is probably the original source of the infectious disease. Outbreaks of Ebola began in 1976 in the Democratic Republic of Congo on the Ebola River, and Sudan, with later outbreaks in Uganda and other West African nations, according to World Health Organization data.

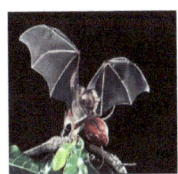 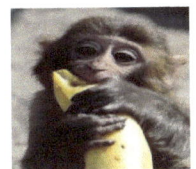 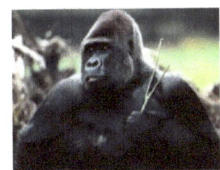

"It is not a casual contact-acquired infection," notes Safdar. Rather, in its later stages, Ebola is passed from person to person via bodily fluids. "There is no known Ebola transmission through coughing or sneezing, like with influenza or tuberculosis," he says. The virus can live on surfaces that are soiled with blood or other body fluids, but sterilizing hospital equipment with bleach kills Ebola viruses."

Symptoms

Early Ebola symptoms are also symptoms of other viral infections. These symptoms include fever, headache, body aches, cough, stomach pain, vomiting, and diarrhea. Because these could be symptoms of other diseases, it's difficult to diagnose Ebola early on. The time it takes from exposure to Ebola to actually getting sick, known as the incubation period, is anywhere from 2 to 21 days, says UAB's Pigott. Most people who are infected with Ebola will develop early symptoms eight to nine days after exposure to the virus. Tests for antibodies against Ebola and viral DNA help doctors make a conclusive diagnosis.

"Later symptoms of Ebola can appear quickly, within a few days after onset of early symptoms. Due to internal and external bleeding, the patient's eyes may become red, and they may vomit blood, have bloody diarrhea, and suffer cardiovascular collapse and death, explains Pigott. The only treatment doctors can provide is supportive care —

they give the patient fluids and oxygen, and keep their blood pressure steady."

FROM US DEPARTMENT

"In order to help people understand some key points about Ebola virus we consulted with our medical specialists at the U S State Department & assembled this list below, worded in plain language for easy understanding.

- The suspected reservoirs for Ebola are fruit bats, monkeys, gorilla, and chimpanzee.
- Transmission to humans is thought to originate from infected bats or chimpanzee, monkeys that have become infected by bats.
- Undercooked infected bat and bush meat transmits the virus to humans.
- Human to human transmission is only achieved by physical contact with a person who is acutely and gravely ill from Ebola virus or their body fluids.
- Transmission among humans is almost exclusively among care-giver, family members or health care workers tending to the very ill. .
- The virus is easily killed by contact with soap, bleach, sunlight, or drying.
- A washing machine will kill the virus in clothing saturated with infected body fluids. .
- A person can incubate the virus without symptoms for 2-21 days, the average being 5-8 days before becoming ill.
- THEY ARE NOT CONTAGIOUS until they are acutely ill. Only when ill does the viral expresses itself first in the blood and other bodily fluids (e.g vomit, feaces, urine, breast milk, semen and sweat). .
- If you are walking around you are not infectious to others.
- There are documented cases from Kikwit, Democratic Republic of Congo of an Ebola outbreak in a village that had the custom of children never touching an ill adult. Children

living for days in one room hut with parents who died from Ebola did not become infected. .

- You can't contact Ebola by handling money or swimming in a pool.
- There's no medical reason to stop flights, close borders, restrict travel or close embassies, businesses or schools.
- Always practice good hand washing techniques,
- You will not contact Ebola if you eat right and do not touch a dying person.
- Please share this information & try not to spread panic on social and other media.

WHAT TO DO WHEN YOU DO NOT WHAT TO DO

Panic and spreading bad news are not the solution to reversing Ebola disease. If you have been looking for easy way to have more energy, prevent and alleviate EBOLA disease and or reverse your other health deteriorating process, do the following:

- Detoxify your body;
- Improve or boost your immune system;
- Avoid killer foods;
- Create radiant health by eating more of healthy (greens) foods.
- When you obey the above, the Ebola disease you hear about today will not come near you, even if you get near to the virus.

Ebola does not have any business with people that obey simple healthy dietary recommendations

EBOLA *Solution Alert*

Hello readers fear not, eat right and Keep to the recommendations above. I promise you will see the salvation of the Lord, for the Ebola diseases you hear about now will not come near you. Now nutritional research is supporting this recommendation. Obey and live. Ebola does not have any business with people that obey simple healthy dietary recommendations.

> You will never find solution for any health challenge, when you search for that solution everywhere EXCEPT where the solution can be found.
> The solution for Ebola is simple...

SEASON ONE
BUILDING HEALTH PROTOCOLS
The Good Health Tool Box

You will never find solution for any challenge, when you search for that solution everywhere except where the solution can be found. *The solution of Ebola is simple...*

People who rely solely upon their Physician for their wellness are often expecting too much. You have to take at least a measure of responsibility for your own health. In the daily task of building and maintaining health, there are many natural tools that can help your need.

The following recommendations are effective tools one can use to build solid foundation for healthy new you.

> People who rely solely upon their Physician for their wellness are often expecting too much. You have to take at least a measure of responsibility for your own health.

Responsibility 1
Detoxification
To Increase Vitality & Energy against Ebola Virus

If you only had one therapy to fight Ebola and for improving health and vitality, what would it be?

Answer: NUTRIENT BASED DETOXIFICATION.

The primary causes of Ebola disease is toxicity and deficiency. Both are a result of not eating right and maintaining healthy lifestyle. If there must be solution for Ebola, there must be the commitment to follow a better and healthier lifestyle. There must be elimination of those foods that contribute to Ebola disease and poor health. There must be drinking of plenty good water and good night rest every day.

Toxicity according Dr. George Malkmus, Founder of Hallelujah Diet, USA, "refers to a level of poisons in the body from foods and *drugs* that have created acidic condition. These poisons are the byproducts of consuming foods from animal sources, as well as sugar, table salt, caffeine and white flour products. These foods also include other foods items that have been altered from their original whole-food designs".

Deficiency is the state we are in when we lack adequate nutrients for the body and is caused by consuming foods that are refined and processed until they are rendered nutritionally

incomplete. In the words of Dr. Chaitow of London England, "a body with healthy immune system, efficient organs of elimination and detoxification, and a sound circulatory and nervous system can handle a great deal of toxicity". But if the body has been damaged by toxicity, deficiency and from chronic exposure to environmental pollutants, (*as we experience everyday*) restoring these functions, organs and systems can only be accomplished through <u>detoxification therapies</u>.

Detoxification accelerates the body's own s natural cleansing processes. This internal cleansing results in toxins/poisons being emptied into the blood stream. Detoxification is a way to cleanse our bodies and rid them of toxins and debris that have accumulated over the years. This gives the body clean foundation upon which the body can build. Just as caring for the car engine, filters, hoses and so forth. Our bodies need maintenance to promote health. Our body's filter is the liver; it needs periodic cleansing.

Through detoxification, we create a good foundation on which to build a stronger body by doing some internal house cleaning. This will include cleansing the body filters, removing the cobwebs and tuning up the engine. The main function of the body is to create homeostasis – a state at which every part of the body is properly balanced and in a state of perfect health.

With the type of lifestyle and dietary choices over the years, the body balance or the homeostasis are upset, the body will begin to malfunction and be in constant mode of repair and restoration, working to keep the body alive at all costs. To achieve healthy living condition, the body tries to rid of the toxic elements that have been forced upon it. If the body fails to fully cleanse itself of the toxins, they may be stored deep within the tissues and cells.

It is when these toxins are stored that the real body damage begins to occur in those areas and signs of disease begin to manifest. At this point, if there is any infectious disease such as Ebola virus, there is likelihood that the body may become victim. This is why cleansing of the body (detoxification) becomes vital and the only way out.

> Just as caring for the car engine, filters, hoses and so forth. Our bodies need maintenance to promote health. Our body's filter is the liver; it needs periodic cleansing.

Why detoxification?

The human body has its own natural way of detoxification. Detoxification is a critical ongoing process for achieving and maintaining health in our body. It involves the elimination of substances which are poisonous and/or for which the body has no further constructive use.

All healthy cells automatically detoxify themselves every day. Up to 80% of all processes of the human body are for detoxification. This means that 80% of a person's physical health picture comes from their ability to efficiently detoxify and eliminate waste, but if the toxins are too much, it needs some help. Nowadays our bodies are exposed to more and more toxic substances - in the **food** we eat, the **water** we drink and **air** we breathe and the materials surrounding us like paints, carpeting, dyes etc. The detoxification Program clears the body toxins which have accumulated over time and overloaded the systems.

> Through detoxification, we create a good foundation on which to build a stronger body by doing some internal house cleaning. This will include cleansing the body filters, removing the cobwebs and tuning up the engine.
> The main function of the body is to create homeostasis – a state at which every part of the body is properly balanced and in a state of perfect health.

The nutritional detoxification formula and personalized diet is designed to take the load off the body's system and give the liver optimal support during this process.

Health Bearing Effect of Toxic Overload

The buildup of toxins in human tissue can impact all body systems. Significant signs of toxic overload include; *fertility issues, Acne, Muscle Weakness, Rashes, Headaches, Fatigue, memory loss, and Depressed Immune Function.* Additionally, low-level, long-term toxic exposure has been linked to chronic conditions such as Parkinson's disease, chronic fatigue syndrome, fibromyalgia syndrome, leukemia, and non-Hodgkin's lymphoma.

The Body's Natural Cleansing Process

The body has natural methods of detoxification. Individual cells get detoxified in the lymph and circulatory system.

Avenues of detoxification

Toxins can be excreted from the body by the liver, kidneys, intestines, the Lymph system, bowels, skin, mucous membrane, and lungs. Detoxification treatments become necessary when the body's natural detoxification systems become overwhelmed.

The Liver

The Liver is the principle organ of detoxification, assisted by the Kidneys and intestines.

The Lymph System

This is part of the immune system, and it assists the body in ridding itself of toxic wastes. The truth is that the lymph does not move through the body unless the body moves. Thus deep breathing and physical exercise are the key elements the lymph uses for detoxification and restoring the immune system.

Mucous Membrane

Drinking adequate amount of water (10–12 glasses) per day will help keep the mucous thin enough to flow out of the body rapidly. The mucous membranes trap toxins and help to move them out of the body; however if the mucous is not kept a thin consistently, the toxins may become trapped and sometimes infection will develop. Drinking adequate water helps a great deal to keep mucous thin.

Bowel Movement

One of the most important issues to address in detoxification is elimination through the bowels. There are some seventy percent people living in Africa, America and Europe who suffer from sluggish bowel movement. This can be a warning sign of greater health problems to come. If dead cells and waste products are not eliminated quickly and properly they can be re absorbed into the body and thus results in a toxic build up. These toxic build ups contribute to the breakdown of the body and illness. To avoid this, it is therefore very vital that bowel function be optimized in order to insure rapid and efficient elimination of toxins and avoid Ebola disease.

The Skin

Elimination through the skin is another avenue of detoxification. This process helps elimination of toxins through dry skin brushing where the dead cells on the skins are brushed away. The human skin is the largest organ in the body and as such when the bowels are not eliminating properly, the toxins will try to get out anyway they can. The skin is one of the avenues.

This explains why some experience rashes, pimples, boils etc. during detoxification. The body is supposed to lose about one kilogram of toxins through the skin daily.

METABOLIC DETOXIFICATION

Everyone knows healing is a process which has many layers. As we peel one layer after another, we can get to the roots of the health issues that have been deeply embedded behind all the daily physical common symptoms such as headaches, intestinal pain, constipation, joint pain, acne, etc.

Metabolic detoxification process helps us get to the roots of the problems by eliminating the superficial layer of symptoms, exposing the causes of illness whether it's some adrenal dysfunction resulting from chronic stress mal-adaptation, thyroid deficiency from an old viral infection, or even some psychological/emotional trauma from a relationship in the past.

Metabolic detoxification process also addresses the whole body, not a single organ or system; thereby restoring biochemical and physiological balances in the body. Metabolic detoxification is a complex process involving a chain of chemical reactions that occur primarily within the liver and kidneys:

Phase I (functionalization): Enzymes secreted by the liver break down toxins into modified, highly reactive molecules. (Ironically, a byproduct of functionalization is the creation of free radicals, molecules that can wreak cellular damage if not quickly neutralized.)

Phase II (conjugation): Chemicals such as the amino acid glutathione produced by the liver bind with the modified toxins, neutralizing them and making them more water soluble.

Transport: Proteins deliver the neutralized toxins to the kidneys, where they are excreted via urine; or the gastrointestinal tract, where they are excreted via the stool.

Optimal metabolic detoxification helps the body cleanse itself of harmful substances before they can accumulate in tissue and affect health. But factors such as toxic overload, genetic predisposition, and insufficient levels of key nutrients can impair this process, increasing a person's susceptibility to toxicity-related diseases.

Metabolic detoxification process also addresses the whole body, not a single organ or system; thereby restoring biochemical and physiological balances in the body. Metabolic detoxification is a complex process involving a chain of chemical reactions that occur primarily within the liver and kidneys:

Responsibility 2
Immune System Boost

Boost the immune system of the body, (*draining the body of the toxins/poisons*); feed the body with nutrient-based living foods, avoid killer foods. The miracle will happen. *Violate these at your own risk...*

Any solution or strategy for Ebola that does not have at its primary goal to boost immune system of the people through what they should and should not eat to produce wellness will fail. It will only produce more physical problems and larger expenditure of money. Almost all sickness and disease have their root causes from lack of strong immune system; improper diet and lifestyle, not necessarily by bacteria, viruses, infection or inheritance as we have been made to believe by media and the industry responsible for medical administration.

The way to restore wellness and provide health solution to the people is to teach how to boost immune system through eating right so as to create wellness. Appropriate public education on health must be one that encourages health and informs that most disease are self-induced by improper diet and lifestyle thus, almost all sickness and disease is preventable by eating right and maintaining healthy lifestyle that produces wellness.

There is this widespread of confidence in the ability of medical science to cure the effects of such life threatening disease once they occur. We think the right information should emphasis the limitations of current practice in curing the common killer diseases such as Ebola and others diseases. Once they occur there is in reality very little that the medical science can do to return the patient to normal physiological function.

> Any solution or strategy for Ebola that does not have at its primary goal to boost immune system of the people through what they should and should not eat to produce wellness will not be sustainable

If the awareness of this limitation is hyped as the life threatening news of Ebola campaign, the importance of prevention will become all the most obvious. As we from this part of the world were taught, and we have come to believed that modern medical technology can solve major health problems while the role of such important factors as *living foods* in cancer and heart disease has long been obscured by the emphasis on the conquest of these diseases through the miracle of modern medicine. Treatment not prevention has been the order of the day. The problem can never be solved only by more and more medical approach.

Our greatest strategy to unlearn what has helped us to create the present problems is to educate the public with the truth. That truth, which is also the greatest medical discovery of our time, is the awesome power within the human body to heal and rejuvenate itself. This tremendous discovery is destined to change the way people practice medicine in our present world. We believe in the near future, instead of drugging the body, cutting the body and working against the natural system of healing, medical practitioners will strive to feed and enhance the body's amazing power of self-healing.

The modern medical community still seems to believe that nutrition cannot prevent disease, and is practically useless in treating it. "Yet we have scientific proof that diet is the single most powerful tool for the treatment of diseases" said Dr. Whiteaker. Yes more powerful than drugs, more powerful than surgery. More powerful than anything in doctors bag. And people can do it by themselves. This idea may look narrow minded to the medical profession to admit but that is the truth we all must know.

Washing of hands with soap, bleach and alcohol; avoiding handshakes and other measures are good but do not guarantee the solution.
If the immune system is weak,

Washing of hands and avoiding handshakes will do little in prevention.

The truth we must know

When people learn and practice the art of eating right and living right, we will have less of the sicknesses that bother us. Nobody will die of Ebola, Cancer, heart diseases, diabetes, high blood pressure because they will be taking measures to prevent them.

The real cause of Ebola is the poisons created in our bodies by the foods we eat and lifestyle we adopted. What the world should do now to prevent Ebola is to eat right to nourish the body well and enable the body eliminate waste products. We were taught that viruses and germs cause Ebola hence we have been studying viruses and germs when we should be studying diet and drainage. The world will be a better place when we understand that the answer has been within ourselves all the time.

You can never find solution for Ebola when you search for the solution everywhere except where the solution can be found. The simple answer for Ebola is simple – drain the body of toxins, feed it properly, and the miracle is done. Violate these at your own risk. Nobody will have Ebola who takes the trouble to avoid it.

Washing hands with soap, bleach and alcohol; avoiding shaking hands and other measures are good but do not guarantee the solution. If the immune system is weak, washing of hands and avoiding handshakes will do little in prevention. Ebola is killing people today because the system is dysfunctional – more expensive, not doing the job of elimination of wastes. Our health care system is in crises. It is geared to provide what is most profitable for the medical community, not what is best for the people of the world. This is what must be stopped if Ebola must stop.

Responsibility 3
Ebola Solution Begins

What we eat and lifestyles we adopt are usually the result of tradition, advertising and habit.

If we begin to make healthy nutrition and lifestyle choices, the body starts the cleansing process – eliminating the bad and putting in the good – and the areas damaged by stored toxins begin to rebuild. The body can often heal itself of many serious physical problems including Ebola. To do this, we must bring conditions that are conducive to healing. This can be done by significantly increasing the nutrition that reaches to the cellular. We must watch what we eat.

Your Diets, Your Lifestyle

What we eat is usually the result of tradition, advertising and habit. I recall the early years of my life; my dietary habit was very similar to those of my parents. As I was growing up, I was introduced to new foods when I left my parents to live on mine own. I associated a lot with friends and colleagues; I also adopted their lifestyle and eating pattern. From this stage I tried new products that came from the markets, including new offerings from fast food eateries. They tasted sweet but before I knew it I incorporated a new item into my diet.

I never knew or seem to realize that what I was putting into my body could have devastating effects. How sad, that I was never taught how to associate what I eat with wellness and healthy lifestyle or my physical, mental and emotional problems. Even though I was ignorant, the truth remains that I literally became what I ate. I now realize that in reality diet and lifestyle influenced my physical life more than any other factor of my life.

It should be noted that Ebola disease was discovered in 1976 and did not become part of West African medical terminology until in the 2010s. Why? What has changed in the past 30 years? What is causing more and more problems in this area with each passing years? In my thinking, I suggest we take a long hard look at the food we have been putting into our bodies and the way we have been living. What can we see? Well, we will find some interesting things including most of the answers to the problems associated with Ebola and other life threatening diseases like cancer, diabetes hypertension etc.

Animal Growth Hormones

Growth hormones in animals were first introduced in United States of America by the meat industry in the 1950s. The essence was to enable farmers get their animals to the market in less time, thus increasing their profits. The success in this marketing strategy motivated Africa and probably other Continents began to copy American strategy as well as the products of the strategy. Little did they realize the significance of this change in the way their meat was being grown.

An example of this would be that chicken from my village in the past took about sixteen to twenty weeks to be ready for the market; now it is ready for market in six weeks due to these growth hormones. The same is applicable to what we call imported frozen chickens. When this chicken is butchered, the growth hormones remain in the flesh of the meat and are consumed at our homes, fast food joints, wedding and birthday parties, as well as in church and political gatherings or conventions.

Now if growth hormones can cause an animal to grow twice or thrice as fast as it normally would grow and cause the chicken to mature in less than half the time designed by God, what do you think these growth hormones will do within our bodies?

Prostate, breast and colon cancers are the fastest growing cancers in Africa today and the primary cause of these cancers is consumption of anima products. The relationship between diets high in animal proteins and cancer has been clearly established. Cancerous cells feed well on animal proteins, which trigger the abnormal proliferation of cells.

According to recent research report, the meat industry has contributed to more deaths in Africa than all the wars of the continent, natural disasters including vehicle accidents combined. Dr. Anderson states that "science used to support the consumption of meat. It no longer does. It cannot. The facts are so overwhelming that the eating of animal sourced foods is doomed as the age of enlightened people is ushered in".

What animal products are doing to the people of the World especially African is a caricature. Today meat products can be linked directly or indirectly to about 80 percent of all physical deaths in Africa. High blood Pressure, Cancer, Ebola, diabetes, strokes are all primarily caused by animal products. Stroke and heart attacks which are killing mostly the rich in Africa today are caused by the clogging of the arteries with fats (cholesterol). It is interesting to note the average animal product consumption in Africa today is putting about 15 kilos of fat into the consumer per year. Animal product is the only source of bad cholesterol.

Prostate, breasts and colon cancers are the fastest growing cancers in Africa today and the primary cause of these cancers is consumption of animal products. The relationship between diets high in animal proteins and cancer has been clearly established. Cancerous cells feed well on animal proteins, which trigger the abnormal proliferation of cells.

Diabetes and high blood pressure continue to take more and more lives in Africa. These killer diseases are becoming more and more prevalent each year. It might be shocker to know that adult onset diabetes is usually not sugar problem, nor a failure of the pancreas to produce enough insulin, but rather a fat problem. The fat coated the cells and prevents the insulin receptor within the cell. Sadly, the high animal protein diet most medical professionals prescribe for their diabetic patients is the very thing that causes diabetes and eventual death.

Research has revealed the primary cause of Ebola is animals – fruit bats, monkeys, chimpanzees, and gorilla including bush meat. We have not been told the truth of what animals and animal products are doing to the people of Africa. And they may not tell us because the animal products industry is paying the bills, providing educational materials for our public schools, sponsoring sports, politics and politicians as well as the professional associations overseeing health and well-being of the people. So it is like saying *Go on... destroy the people*.

Finally on the growth hormones in meat, one of the most horrible effects of these artificial growth hormones is what they are doing to our young girls. According to Google search "growth hormones in meat are made of synthetic estrogen, similar to a hormone that is naturally produced in small amounts in a woman's body. Synthetic estrogen has been found to cause numerous problems, including cancer and emotional imbalances. Estrogen is the hormone in its natural form that God designed females to start producing in their bodies at the age of 15 to 16 years. This is what initiates puberty.

If you look at the age of puberty some 20 and 30 years ago, it was usually in the same range of 15 and 16 years. Today, what are we experiencing? Our young girls start their menstrual cycle at the age of 10, 11, 12 years on the average and some even earlier. Can you imagine the monumental problem we are facing as our young girls reproducing at tender age? These come with socio-economic and physical challenges. Our foods and lifestyle is creating health problems. In ignorance we have adopted the unhealthy foods and lifestyle hence we are experiencing the consequences.

FOODS TO AVOID –
(Secret of Overcoming Ebola)

Animal products

Inorganically produced animal sourced foods including fish; this will enable the body to have few complications to deal with. By eliminating the animal products, artificial hormones are also eliminated. Animal products especially flesh is primary cause of bone diseases (osteoporosis) as they create an acidic conditions within the body. This acidity causes the body to remove the calcium from the bones in an effort to neutralize the acidity. We have also found that almost all those infected with Ebola consume large amounts of meat. They were infected because the meat in them weakened their immunity to fight external aggression.

Table Salt

Whoever that recommended that table salt can prevent Ebola is uninformed. When we add table salt to our meals, we create many problems within our body; including high blood pressure and water retention. In the family where animal products and table salts are not consumed, they can never be infected by Ebola virus.

To keep Ebola away from you avoid all processed foods. This may interest you to add to your knowledge. After the food manufacturers have destroyed almost all nutritional value during food processing, they always add salt and sugar. Why? Because without these additions, there is practically no food products on our today's supermarket shelf that would pass the taste, and thus no one would buy their products. Our bodies receive all the natural sodium they need from fresh and raw vegetables and fruits. In those processed food products on the shelf of supermarkets contain practically zero nutrition.

Sugar

Sugar immobilizes our immune system. Just a bottle of soft drink contains about 9 teaspoon of sugar… enough to immobilize the immune system by 8 hour of the day. Sugar causes the pancreases to malfunction leading to hypoglycemia and moods swing. Sugar depletes the body reserve of vitamin B and other Vitamins and minerals.

If you look at the age of puberty some 20 and 30 years ago, it was usually in the same range of 15 and 16 years. Today, what are we experiencing? Our young girls start their menstrual cycle at the age of 10, 11, 12 years on the average and some even earlier. Can you imagine the monumental problem we are facing as our young girls reproducing at tender age?

Responsibility 4
Overcoming
EBOLA Disease
Fear Not – Create Radiant Healthy Lifestyle

A strong immune system is paramount for Ebola prevention and survival. With a mortality rate ranging from 50 to 80 percent, Ebola is a virus nobody would ever want to meet.

Are you not afraid of Ebola? A participant asked me after "THOU SHALL NOT BE AFRAID OF EBOLA" Health Seminar I presented at Good Health Center. In my response, I said, people around the world are now concerned, watching the devastating effect the Ebola outbreak has had on those who have come in contact with it. And if not properly managed, Ebola could without doubt be the most destructive disease the world has ever faced in years. I said this because, while Ebola virus seems to be mostly contained to some West African countries, its destructive effect could quickly be a global effect. It was a flight by just one person from Liberia to Nigeria that brought Ebola pandemic to Nigeria. In just few days Ebola become a burning issue in Nigeria.

A strong immune system is paramount for Ebola prevention and survival. With a mortality rate ranging from 50 to 80 percent, Ebola is a virus nobody would ever want to meet. Currently, we are told, there is no available vaccine for this virus, no cure and no medical treatment that has proven to be effective against Ebola virus. This means Ebola can wipe out entire community and could also cause the entire city to live in fear. Victims' isolation and avoidance of contact is the only recommendation as the way to stop the Ebola virus for now.

Ebola virus spreads like HIV virus, except that the Ebola viral infection is highly contagious and can rapidly kill victims. Only one to eight virus particles are enough to cause an infection in a person. Common prevention strategy demands for avoiding direct contact and airborne droplets of the body fluids. As stated earlier, Ebola virus, during an acute phase of infection, is present in the blood, saliva, stool, semen, breast milk and other bodily fluid containing blood due to hemorrhaging. There is no proving that causal contact with a person's skin can pass the infection.

> While Ebola virus seems to be mostly contained to some West African countries, it destructive effect could quickly be of global effect. It was a flight by just one person from Liberia to Nigeria that brought Ebola pandemic to Nigeria. In just few days Ebola become a burning issue in Nigeria causing the Government millions of Dollars.

I am in agreement with the general recommendation that quarantine and isolation is to prevent the spread of the Ebola virus or any other virus in same deadly category. However when quarantine and isolation has already failed, there are natural products that can help your immune system from being depleted when you face an Ebola viral attack.

There are basic food components that have proven excellent for immune system support when dealing with Ebola virus and similar viruses. Please note that these immune system support foods are not being offered to people to treat, cure, prevent or alleviate Ebola diseases by themselves. These only provide excellent supports for the God given abilities of the immune system to conquer any infection it is presented with, when properly and adequately supported.

Ebola is a strong infection; therefore it requires strong immune system. Ebola has claimed many lives in Africa because the people underestimated the depletion of the immune system caused by Ebola infection hence we also underestimate the amount of support that is required to mount strong and sufficient immune response.

For strong and sufficient immune system support when dealing with Ebola virus, we must understand that the body has a God-given, built-in-ability to heal itself and that the role of the physician is to aid or enhance this process with natural therapies such as vitamins and minerals derived from living foods – (vegetables fruits, nuts, seeds, herbs).

THE VITAMINS

In health and disease management, vitamins are important. They perform vital and specific roles in the body chemistry. They are like electric sparks which helps to run human motors. It is not possible to sustain life without all the essential vitamins. Except for a few exceptions, vitamins cannot be manufactured or synthesized. The absence or improper absorption of vitamins results in specific deficiency. All Ebola victims are vital vitamin deficient. Vitamins must be in their natural state and they are found in minute quantities in organic foods. We must obtain them from natural foods or in dietary supplements.

Vitamins are potent organic compounds which are found in small concentrations in foods. They are of immense help in fighting diseases and speeding recovery. They perform dual purposes in health management - Correcting deficiencies and treating diseases in place of drugs. Vitamins are of several kinds; differ from each other in physiological functions, in chemical structure and in their distribution in food. They are also broadly divided into two categories namely fat soluble and water soluble.

Vitamins A, D, E and K are all soluble in fat and fat solvent and therefore known as fat soluble. The vitamin B-Complex and Vitamin C are water soluble. They dissolve easily in water. A portion of these Vitamins may actually be destroyed by heating. They cannot be stored in the body hence they have to be taken daily in food. Any extra quantity taken in any one day is eliminated as waste.

Please note that these immune system support foods are not being offered to people to treat, cure, prevent or alleviate Ebola diseases by themselves. These only provide excellent supports for the God given abilities of the immune system to conquer any infection it is presented with, when properly an adequately supported.

THE MINERALS

Minerals are vital to health. Like vitamins and amino acids, mineral are essential for regulating and building the trillions of living cells which make up the body. Each of the body cell receives the essential food element through the blood streams. They must therefore be properly nourished with adequate supply of all the essential minerals for the efficient functioning of the body. Minerals help maintain the volume of water necessary for life process in the body. They help draw chemical substances into and out of the cells and keep the blood and tissue fluid from becoming either too acidic or too alkaline.

The importance of minerals in the body just like vitamins can be illustrated by the fact that there over 30,000 enzymes in the body which direct growth and energy. Each enzyme has minerals and vitamins associated to it. The minerals and vitamin elements needed to fight Ebola are Selenium, Iodine and Vitamin C, etc. These are helpful to mount an effective immune response and they can be for additive and possible synergetic healing effect as well.

Selenium

According to Donaldson Michael PhD, a US based Senior Research Fellow "Selenium is very important for the activity of the antioxidant enzyme glutathione peroxidase and it plays vital role in our immune system. Selenium is the mineral element responsible for the prevention of blood clotting reaction. As severe deficiency of Selenium causes blood clotting leading to hemorrhaging.

A reaction observed in animals infected with hemorrhagic viruses. Though we do not have a lot of experience with Ebola virus, many lessons can be learned from RNA virus and HIV virus. Both of these viruses transform quickly because there is not as much translational error-checking with RNA as there is with DNA.

It has been discovered that RNA and HIV viruses thrive is selenium deficient areas of West African region. When the infected person has a high selenium status, as well as an overall antioxidant state, viral replication is slowed, but when selenium

is low or deficient, it causes the virus to multiply furiously, and also causes more mutation leading to more virulent strains. The selenium status of the infected person affects the outcome of the viral infection. This effect may be direct on the virus as well as indirect effects via strengthening the immune system.

Food Sources for Selenium
This mineral is found in Brewer's yeast, garlic, onions, tomatoes etc.

Iodine

Iodine, in the correct molecular form, has properties similar to chlorine, being in the same chemical column in the periodic table. Iodide and chloride are fairly inert. But hypoiodite and hypochlorite solutions are very good sanitizers, anti-viral, anti-parasitic, anti-bacterial, anti-germ substances. Bleach is a well-known germ killer. But you cannot take bleach internally because it is too caustic and destructive. However, iodine can be taken internally without the biological destruction of bleach, but with the same sort of germicidal properties. This is why surgeons wash with iodine substances, and skin is cleansed with iodine preparations before surgery. It kills germ without damaging skin.

Iodine has been known to be used by white blood cells (leukocytes) to kill bacteria for nearly 50 years. Leukocytes use their peroxidase enzyme, combined with hydrogen peroxide and iodine to kill bacteria. This is a normal function of iodine in the body. More recently, a special form of iodine, *nascent iodine*, was shown to be particularly useful in strengthening the immune response to malaria. A simple treatment regimen of nascent iodine enabled people's immune systems to successfully fight off the malaria parasite.

While all iodine has some of these germicidal properties, only nascent iodine excels in supplying iodine that the immune system readily utilizes. Though the properties of nascent iodine have been known for decades, it has been difficult to produce true and stable nascent iodine. Iodine normally exists in nature in a dimer state as diatomic iodine; it also can be combined with potassium or sodium to form the common ionic form. In a novel patented treatment, using an intense electromagnetic field, iodine molecules, can be teased apart into singlet iodine. Iodine is not usually stable in this singlet form, which is why a lot of energy is required to produce this magnetically charged form of iodine. This singlet iodine is called nascent iodine, and it is the form of iodine that will give you the help you need to support a vigorous immune system response to a strong viral infection.

There are a few different manufacturers of nascent iodine as well. The nascent iodine that Hallelujah Diet sells is exactly the same product that provided efficacious immune system support in the clinical trial in India. This nascent iodine is the real thing, and you don't want to take chances on a product that might work when dealing with an Ebola viral infection. You want one that has proven protection—Nascent Iodine from Hallelujah Diet.

Food Sources for iodine

The best dietary sources of iodine are kelp and other seaweeds. Other good sources are turnip greens, garlic, watercress, pineapples, pears, artichokes, citrus fruits and fish liver oils.

Vitamin C

Vitamin C prevents and cures infections effectively, neutralizes various toxins in the system, speeds healing processes in virtually all cases of ill health, increases sexual vitality and

prevents premature ageing. According to Dr. Linus Pauling, a world famous chemist and nutrition expert, "because vitamin C is one of the least toxic vitamins, it is very safe to use in high doses." Your body will take exactly what it needs and excrete any excess naturally."

In a recent paper presented by Dr. Michael on Ebola virus, he said "One important note about the Ebola viral infection is that it induces a very acute case of scurvy, which leads to internal and external bleeding. When all of the vitamin C and antioxidants has been used up in the body, there are none left to maintain the integrity of the blood vessels. This mechanism, coupled with the severe selenium deficiency discussed above, which causes clots to form in capillaries, raises the local blood pressure and puts excessive strain on the weakened vessel walls. So, massive bleeding ensues. Providing vitamin C and other antioxidants is a very important aspect of overcoming an Ebola infection. There is a new oral form of vitamin C called liposomal vitamin C that is proving very effective at replenishing the body's depleted stores of vitamin C.

Dr. Thomas Levy, MD, JD who literally wrote the book on vitamin C and infectious diseases has worked extensively with both intravenous vitamin C and liposomal vitamin C. He was skeptical initially at the results from liposomal vitamin C, but the great results convinced him that liposomal vitamin C was a very powerful product. In a lecture he said, "I proved to my satisfaction that 5-6 grams of properly encapsulated liposomal vitamin C taken orally had a greater clinical impact than a 50 gram infusion." He gave a case report of a 15 year old girl in Colombia with hemorrhagic Dengue fever. She made a remarkable recovery when given 10 grams of liposomal vitamin C over a 24-hour period. This is certainly a relevant case report of the immune-boosting properties when discussing hemorrhagic Ebola fever. Liposomal vitamin C provides strong support for the immune system when dealing with hemorrhagic fever.

Food Sources for Vitamin C

This vitamin is found in citrus fruits, berries, green and leafy vegetables, tomatoes, potatoes and green grams.

Responsibility 5
Oxygen and Exercise
Secret of Overcoming Ebola

The greatest need of the body to overcome Ebola is pure air. Because approximately 90 percent of man's nutritional need comes from the air while the rest from the food we eat.

Not too long ago, I visited a funeral home and looked into the open casket. I saw the motionless and lifeless body of my friend's dad who was about to be committed to the mother earth. While my friend, his family members and all of us the well-wishers, were sorrowful over the departed, I looked into the casket and saw the motionless and lifeless body, I had deep inspiration. I asked myself "what makes man motionless and lifeless? What is the difference between this man in the casket and others walking about, who have come to honor him in death?

While these thoughts were going on in my mind, the preacher's voice came up loud through the mounted speakers and distracted my thoughts. He quoted Genesis 2:7 *"And the Lord God formed man of the dust of the ground and breathed into his nostrils the breath of life and man became a living soul"*. Then he continued God made man with two major raw materials, *the dust of the ground and the breath of life.*

The dust of thy ground

When God formed man of the dust of the ground, God had nothing but a lifeless body, similar to what we are seeing here. (Referring to the body in casket) At death, when a body is placed in the ground; it eventually reduces to the same ingredients from which man was originally made from - the dust of the ground.

OXYGEN - The Breath of Life

Addressing the second component in the raw materials revealed to me the most basic and important substance in man. The raw material is of great importance that without it life in absolutely and positively impossible. Brethren; the preacher said, the substance I am talking about is the *breath of God* which in our today's understanding the **oxygen**. I adjusted my ear to grab what the preacher was saying.

The big question I asked myself; could it be that God breathed into Adam the breath of life (oxygen according to the preacher) that the dead heap of minerals and vitamins sprang to life? Can we say just as oxygen was absolutely necessary to produce life in Adam, it is the same oxygen that is absolutely important to sustain life in today's man?

As those words were hitting my ears, I placed my right hand on my chest to feel the soft and automatic rising and falling as air enters into and exits from my lung. I imagined without the intake of air (oxygen) our physical body would lie lifeless as my friend's dad inside the casket.

The preacher's voice was adjusted for his audience to understand the next illustration. He said at birth when a child comes from the womb its first and most important need to live is not food or water but air. The baby takes into its little body that first breath and immediately we see the chest start to rise and fall and continues till he grows into adult and old age. This rising is taking in of oxygen and falling of the chest is the lung giving off carbon dioxide.

Importance of Oxygen

If we are to cut off oxygen supply for few moments; we would become equally aware of our need for oxygen – (*the life giving and life sustaining substance*). Have you ever find yourself in a smoke filled room, you will automatically and rapidly seek fresh air as the body expresses urgent need for oxygen for the body. If the body is unable to obtain fresh air, that body soon suffocates to death.

To understand the importance of oxygen we must first realize that the human body is a living organism, comprised of about 100 trillion cells. Each cell is capable of reproducing itself. But for the cell to reproduce itself, there are basic needs that must be met. The cell must be fed adequately with an efficient waste disposal system. The adequate

supply of food and efficient waste disposal system determines the quality and length of our lives.

What happens to people that smoke? Those that smoke slowly and surely cut off their oxygen supply as the tars in the smoke coat their lungs. These coatings at the lungs restrict the intake of oxygen and the person slowly and surely suffocates the body cells, depriving them of their most important nutritional need.

Tobacco smoke contains carbon monoxide, the same deadly substance found in vehicle exhaust pipes. What carbon monoxide does in the body is it combines with the hemoglobin in the blood and further reduces its oxygen carrying capacity says Dr. Festus.

This oxygen decrease causes the heart to pump faster to try to make up for the shortage, restricts the blood vessel thereby creating poor circulation.

To understand the importance of oxygen we must first realize that the human body is a living organism, comprised of about 100 trillion cells. Each cell is capable of reproducing itself. But for the cell to reproduce itself, there are basic needs that must be met. The cell must be fed adequately with an efficient waste disposal system. The adequate supply of food and efficient waste disposal system determines the quality and length of our lives.

> Doctors and various African Governments have told us that Ebola and other terminal diseases have no cure. This also means the millions dollars being pumped in the fight against Ebola will be of no permanent and sustainable effect.

Sicknesses in the body manifest in different forms. Ebola, diabetes, headaches, arthritis, and heart attacks are as result of the failure to provide the cells with proper building materials and/or failing to adequately remove the wastes from the cells. This also means improper diet and lifestyle are main causes of sicknesses.

Sadly our society has been programmed into thinking differently. We neglect the basic needs of our body - adequate supply of nutrient filled foods and efficient waste disposal system. When our body begins to manifest sickness, we reach out for miracle drugs. Doctors and governments have told us that Ebola and other terminal diseases have no cure. This also means the millions governments are pumping in the fight against Ebola will be of no permanent and sustainable effect.

If anybody wants to know the secret of over overcoming Ebola he or she must take control of his health and observe the natural laws as given by God the maker of man. If we do that Ebola will not come in first place. In most instances, when we eliminate the causes of our physical problems, give the body the proper and well-nourished food, healing will come naturally and rapidly too.

But in all these, what is the relationship of oxygen in overcoming Ebola. We have established that the greatest need of man is oxygen. Now let us consider other facts about oxygen in the fight against Ebola. The quality of air we breathe affects the quality and life we live. Breathing polluted air decreases the quality and length of life. Increase supply of oxygen makes the body to be

full of energy and life. Decreased supply of oxygen to the cells makes the body to fail to provide the required energy for proper functioning thereby forcing the body to feel tired and sluggish. Increased supply of oxygen to the body will prevent Ebola and other sicknesses to have foothold while the insufficient supply of the oxygen make the body a breeding ground for sickness including Ebola.

How to oxygenate the body

Eating living food is the starting point because most people's miseries begin by eating the wrong foods. Living foods will start to normalize body weight and increase energy. Increased energy demand free breathing flow and deep breathing enhances free breathing and larger intake of oxygen by the body. Increase oxygen oxygenates and stimulates the cells and thus produce superior health. The next thing the body needs is exercising

> If anybody wants to know the secret of over overcoming Ebola he or she must take control of his health and observe the natural laws as given by God, the maker of man. If we do that Ebola will not come in first place. In most instances, when we eliminate the causes of our physical problems, give the body the proper and well-nourished food, healing will come naturally and rapidly too.

EXERCISE IN HEALTH AND DISEASE

A world famous physical educationist, Eugene Sandow, "*Life is movement; stagnation is death*" Physical exercise is essential for the maintenance of normal condition of life. Lack of natural exercise is one of the chief causes of weakness and ill-health. In recent years, the need for exercise has been recognized even in sickness. Physio and occupational therapy are now standard procedures in medicine to restore the use of muscles and nerves that have been injured by disease or by accident.

> The less active persons ran a three times higher risk of suffering a fatal heart attack than did those who worked the hardest. Review of fatal heart attacks revealed that the less

> active men were also three times more likely to die unexpectedly and rapidly within an hour after the attack.

Exercise and Activity

For corrective living, it is essential to differentiate between *exercise* and *activity*. While both are important as they are involved in vital physical movement, they vary in degree and benefits. Both employ the body in voluntary movement.

<u>Exercise</u> employs the body over the widest possible range of movement for the particular purpose of maintaining or acquiring muscle tone and control with maximum joint flexibility. Exercise demands considerable physical effort and is more beneficial as mental concentration is simultaneously employed.

<u>Activity</u> uses the body to a limited degree and generally to achieve a specific purpose. Activity requires less physical effort and often less conscious effort once the routine has been established.

Benefits

A strong connection between a hard and a healthy hard has also been convincingly demonstrated in a recent study. The study showed that the less active persons ran a three times higher risk of suffering a fatal heart attack than did those who worked the hardest. Review of fatal heart attacks revealed that the less active men were also three times more likely to die unexpectedly and rapidly within an hour after the attack.

Systematic physical exercise has many benefits. The more important benefits are mentioned below:

- Improved capillary action in the working of muscular and brain tissue results from exercise carried to the point of real endurance. This permits greater blood flow and gives the muscles, including the heart, more resistance to fatigue. Massage, heat and moderate exercise are relatively ineffective in producing additional capillary action as compared with vigorous exercise. The full use of the lungs in vigorous exercise can reduce or prevent lung congestion due to lymph accumulation.
- Better respiratory reserve is developed by persistent exercise. This ensures better breath holding, especially after a standard exercise. With greater respiratory reserves, exercise becomes easier.
- Regular exercise taken properly can achieve the increased use of food by the body which contributes to health and fitness. The basal metabolic rate and habitual body temperature will slowly rise during several weeks of physical exercise, if the program is

not too hard. The healthy person usually has abundant body heat and a warm radiant glow.

- Regular exercise plays an important role in the fight against stress. It provides recreation and mental relaxation besides keeping the body physically and mentally fit. It is nature's best tranquillizer.
- Chronic fatigue caused by poor circulation can be remedied by undertaking some exercise on a daily basis. It helps relieve tension and induces sleep. Moderate physical exercise at the end of a try day can bring a degree of freshness and renewed energy.
- Gas and intra-intestinal accumulations can be reduced by exercise that acts to knead and squeeze or vibrate the intra-intestinal mass.
- Improvement in tone and function of veins can be accomplished by repetitiously squeezing and draining the blood out of them and then allowing them to fill.
- Sweating in exercise aids kidneys by helping to eliminate the waste matter from the body. Consistent exercise leads to improvement in quality of blood. Studies have shown
- Improved hemoglobin levels, relatively greater alkalinity, improved total protein content and a grater red cell count.
- Systemic exercise promotes physical strength and mental vigor and strengthens will power and self-

control leading to harmonious development of the whole system.

Methods of Exercise

Several systems of exercise have been developed over the years. Whichever system you choose to adopt, the exercises should be performed systematically, regularly and under proper guidance.

The best way to accomplish this is by:

Walking

Deep breathing,

Aerobic

The minimum amount of exercise recommended is 20 minutes every day

Final shot

Do you seek to take responsibility for your state of well-being and health? You want to live healthy and without sickness. if your answer is yes, then boost your immune system and maintain healthy living.

www.ingramcontent.com/pod-product-compliance
Lightning Source LLC
Chambersburg PA
CBHW050828290526
45792CB00001B/306